ALPHA OMEGA YOGA

ALPHA OMEGA YOGA

The Art and Science of
Self Transformation

Written and Illustrated by

Angela Kolias

Library of Congress Control Number: 2011905885
ISBN: Hardcover   978-1-4628-5631-2
                Softcover   978-1-4628-5630-5
                Ebook   978-1-4628-5632-9

This book was printed in the United States of America.

To order additional copies of this book, contact:
Xlibris Corporation
1-888-795-4274
www.Xlibris.com
Orders@Xlibris.com
96339

For our big, fat human family—
with love, light, and joy.

Contents

Illustrations

The art of life is the most distinguished
and rarest of all the arts.

—Carl Gustav Jung,
Modern Man in Search of a Soul

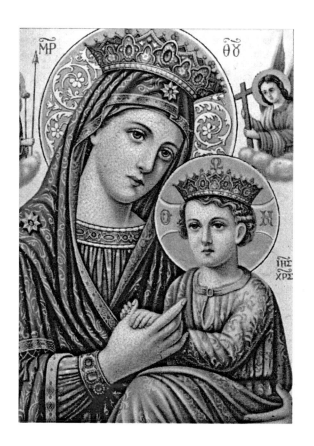

Our own personal tragedies can make us
poets or demons,
spiritual giants, or emotional vampires . . .
If only we could understand and learn from them.

Sometimes, we need to actually appreciate our tragedies
and use them as vehicles toward a greater humanity.
If we live with them in a positive manner,
we can even learn to be "healers."

Tragedies there be for everyone—some lesser, some
greater—but the one who learns to increase in spirit and
humanity from them is a gift to mankind.

—Orthodox archbishop Lazar Puhalo

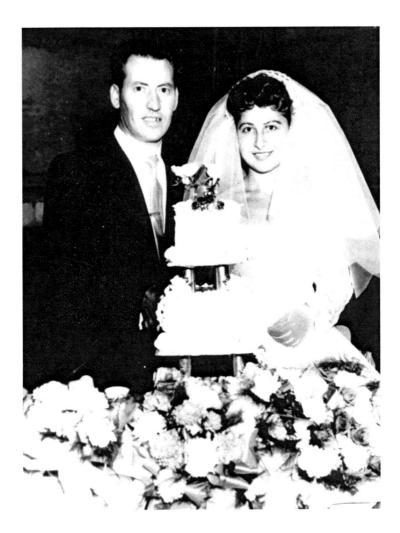

My parents Gust and Nina Kolias—August 21, 1959

Introduction

My father said that life is a tragedy and a catastrophe
and that we have a choice whether to laugh or cry.
Mostly I have chosen to laugh,
but God/dess knows,
I have also cried plenty.

My mother came to Canada to marry my father never
having met him but by photograph and letter of reference.
She raised her four children, constantly proclaiming in
Greek, "Then xero ti na sas po pedia!
O Theos na sas fotisi!"
"I do not know what to tell you children!
May God enlighten you!"
Her prayers worked.

This book is the result of half a century of
study and practice.

In the Greek culture, we wish people a lifetime of
one hundred years: "Na ta ekatostisis."
This means I am now half done with my life here.

I now look forward to spending the second half of my life
sharing with my big, fat human family the knowledge and
experience I have come by on my path of enlightenment.

My approach has been to seek the underlying unity of
wisdom and to articulate it as simply as possible.

My father and the Buddha have it right. Life is suffering!
But life is also a miracle!

Before enlightenment—
chop wood, boil water, make tea . . .

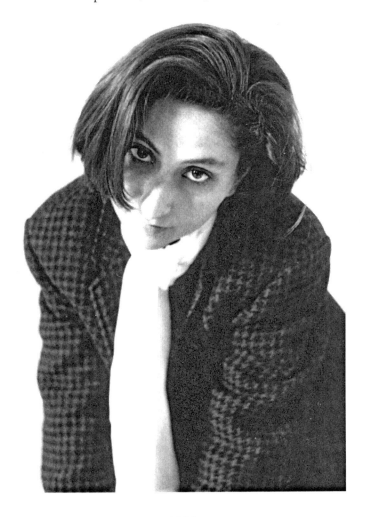

■1985■

After enlightenment—
chop wood, boil water, make tea . . .

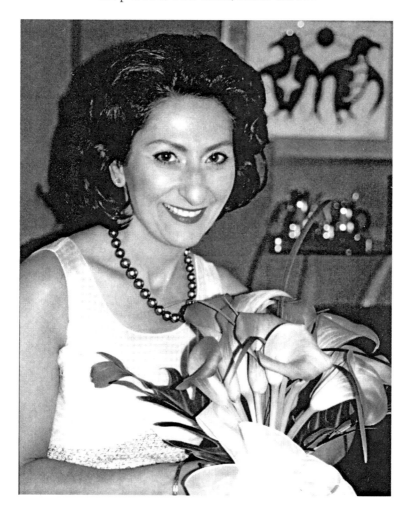

♦2005♦

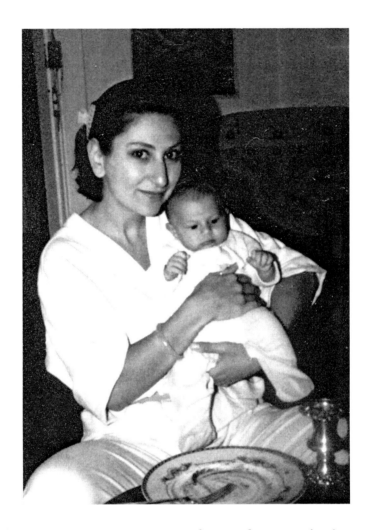

This poem was written summer of 1985 after giving birth to my
daughter, Sheika Luna Sol at home on my own.

Birth-Death-Enlightenment

In search of God,
I turned within.

"You are strong and intelligent,"
my ego told me.

So I swam to the bottom
of my guts
and discovered
weakness.

The Human Condition:

We are all but babes—
born in blood,
destined to die.

Our first cries
live on within.

Life, insecure and vulnerable, unfolds,
and we see

The only "Real Thing"
in Relativity
is "RelationShip."

The world as I knew it has crumbled.

Now I AM
in the middle of Nowhere,
holding
Divine Mother's Hand.

And finally
I have the courage to

LOVE.

Birth

The Unified Universe,
Infinite and Conscious,
spirals through the dimensions.

Through the gateway
of the Womb,
a baby is born
into the fabric
of time and space.

Some babies remain conscious

of their cosmic journey
as they fall to earth,

but most do not.

Thus, Ignorance begins.

We each appear as a distinct individual—
a human self which in Greek is known as "ego."
"Ego" simply means "I" or "me."

Because we are now in relativity,
we are no longer One.

The ONE has become two,
and the two have become the many.

The Universe
has given birth.

Welcome to physical manifestation.

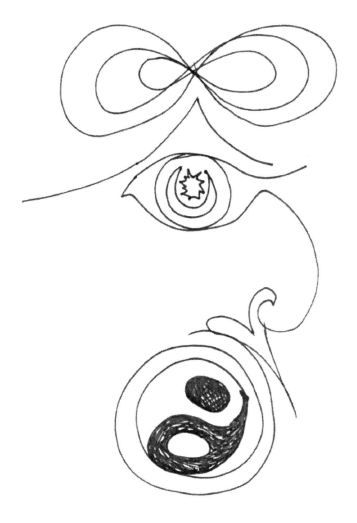

It is a riddle wrapped in a mystery inside an enigma.

—Winston Churchill

Relationships

It is a Mystery why

the Infinite Universe,
in order to know Itself,
entered into Duality.

Relative Reality appeared, and
as human Beings, we are now a part of this picture.

As babies, our primary relationship is with
the Mother.

Some earthly mothers are healthy and loving
toward their children,
and some are not.

Some earthly mothers are loved and supported
by their mates,
and some are not.

Being human in relationship is challenging,
but it does not stop our deepest desire—
to Be
in community
with someone to Love and
with someone who Loves us.

Where can we cling?

Where can we find safety?

How do we find our Beloved?

Thus begins the journey
back
to
Knowledge.

KNOW THYSELF.

Who are we?

Why are we here?

What are we supposed to be doing here?

There is a name for the fairy tale.

It is called "Ayios Gamos,"

the Mystical Marriage.

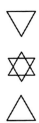

Union
"Ayios Gamos"
The Mystical Marriage

Yoga,

which simply means

"Union"

to unite,

is about uniting with the Divine.

Becoming One—

whole,
holy.

Transcending duality,
re-entering Cosmic Consciousness.

Integrated.

Liberated.

Enlightened.

As humans, we use tools
of warp and weft
to try and understand
that which is beyond the
veil of space and time.

Concepts can help.

"Offering ourselves up to God."
"Children of Divine Mother."
"Brides of Christ."
"Instruments of the Holy Spirit."

Concepts can also hurt.

Because Infinity cannot be named,
Infinity cannot be boxed or packaged.
Not by any religion.
Not by any philosophy.

But it can be
experienced.

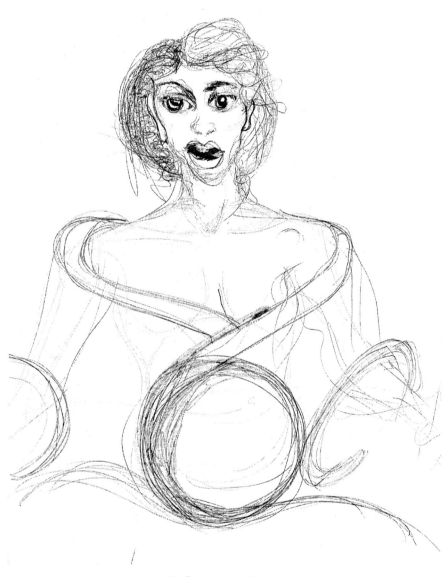

Infinity Breathing
Self portrait 1985

Experience
Yoga Practice

The spiritual alchemy of transformation

begins
with the instrument
we have at hand—

our body.

The physical practice of
Yoga

consists of

Asana,
which means posture,

and
Pranayama,
the observance of the life-giving Breath.

Prana
means "Life Force,"
"Chi," or "Qi"
Inspiration
in Spirit
and even "Holy Spirit."

The practice
of
proper alignment (Asana/Posture)
and breath (Pranayama)

opens
our inner space,

dissolves
our barriers,

allows
the Infinite Life Force
to
breathe (through) us.

Aligned
with cosmic forces,
our body
becomes

a Divine Instrument
receiving,
reflecting,
radiating

Divine Light.

I am created by Divine Light.
I am sustained by Divine Light.
I am protected by Divine Light.
I am surrounded by Divine Light.
I am ever growing into Divine Light.

—Swami Sivanada Radha.

The Divine Light Invocation:
 a healing meditation.

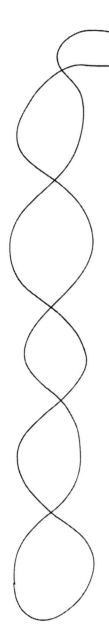

Awareness and Alignment

Where does the mind end and
the body begin?

Where does the body end and
the mind begin?

The brain
is like a crystal
a liquid crystal

a receiving and transmitting station

with the spine
as the central axis.

Which channel to tune into?

The Ultimate Reality Show.
The Alpha and the Omega.
The Divine.

Awareness and Alignment
allow us to
tune in
to the frequency
and to
tune out
the static.

Learning to relax is key.

Releasing the tension
held in our body and mind
that blocks the flow,

realigning our bones,

creating space
where
body, breath, and consciousness
(body, mind, and spirit)

All
Come
Together,

Opening
our
energy
channels
to
a
state
of

Grace.

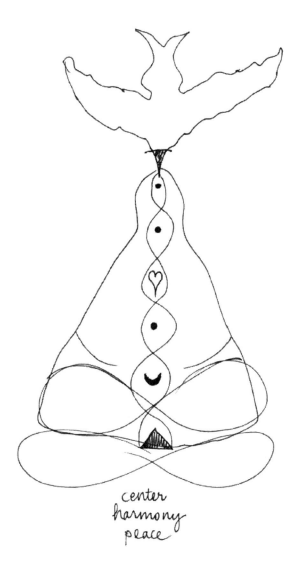

center
harmony
peace

Before speaking or acting, take time to find your center.

—Zen saying

If there is harmony in the home,
there will be order in the nation.

If there is harmony in the nation,
there will be peace in the world.

—The Tao

Relaxing, Releasing, Realigning

Learning to Die
is where to begin.

Savasana,
which means
"posture of the corpse,"
is about
letting go
and letting God in,

surrendering body back
to Mother Earth's support,

laying bones long
through both ends
with shoulder blades rolled down.

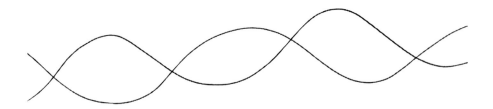

Jaw loose,
sigh,

AOM.

Throat open and hollow
to the golden silence.

Eyes soft in their sockets,
forehead and eyebrow smooth
that the third eye
may awaken.

Dome of the skull
opens it oculus,

allowing Light to enter,
flooding the emptiness of our body
now ready for

Life.

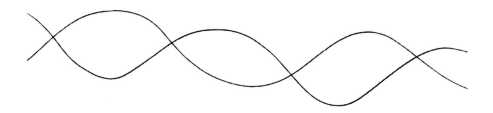

SAVASANA

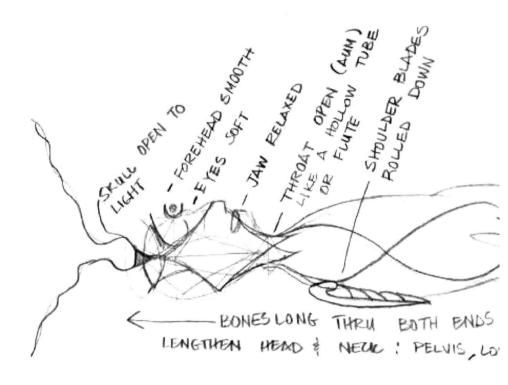

SKULL OPEN TO LIGHT
– FOREHEAD SMOOTH
– EYES SOFT
JAW RELAXED
THROAT OPEN (AUM) LIKE A HOLLOW TUBE OR FLUTE
SHOULDER BLADES ROLLED DOWN

← BONES LONG THRU BOTH ENDS
LENGTHEN HEAD & NECK : PELVIS, LO'

RELAXING
SURRENDERING
TO THE BREATH
THAT INFINITE LIFE FORCE
MAY FILL & FLOW
THROUGH THE BODY

`CORPSE POSE`

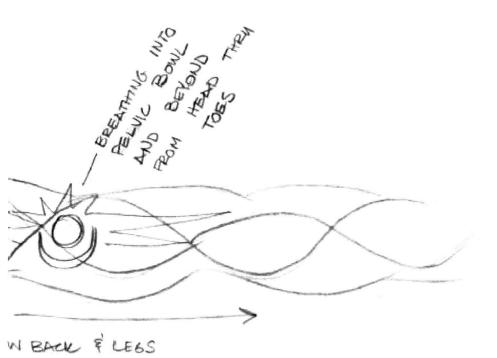

BREATHING INTO PELVIC BOWL AND BEYOND FROM HEAD THRU TOES

W BACK & LEGS

BREATH FLOWS FREELY
TO AND FRO
FROM HEAD THROUGH TOES
LETTING GO INTO EMPTINESS
IN ORDER TO RECEIVE
PRANA, DIVINE LIGHT, HOLY SPIRIT

My true religion is kindness.

—the fourteenth Dalai Lama

Humility is truly the mother of all virtues.
It makes us a vessel, a vehicle, an agent
instead of "the source" of the principal.
It unleashes all other learning, all growth and process.

—Stephen Covey

Life in the Body

Peeling away the layers of illusion
to get to the core
of
Emptiness,

that we may be filled
with
the Infinite Divine Force.

Humility—
which in Greek means "being
down to and of the earth"—

begins by surrendering
unnecessary attitude
from our face and body.

Buddha face serenely smiling—the inner smile
soft eyes/smooth forehead, relaxed jaw/hollow throat—

opens
the "bottleneck"
into a gateway,

that we may invite
Holy Spirit
to physically enter
within.

The Breath of Holy Spirit
plays (with) us
like a flute—a wind instrument
protecting us,
directing us,
sustaining and surrounding us.

With every breath we take,
with every step we make,

we are not alone.

Thank God/dess.

BUDDHA FACE SERENELY SMILING

FOREHEAD
SMOOTH ——

EYES SOFT IN SOCKETS ——

JAW RELAXED, RELEASED ——

DROP THE CHIN ——

DISENGAGE THE LARYNX
INTO A SIGH ——
A SILENT "AUM"
THAT THROAT BECOMES
AN OPEN TUBE BETWEEN
MIND & BODY

KEEP VERTABRAES OF NECK -
LONG (LENGHTEN BACK OF
NECK)

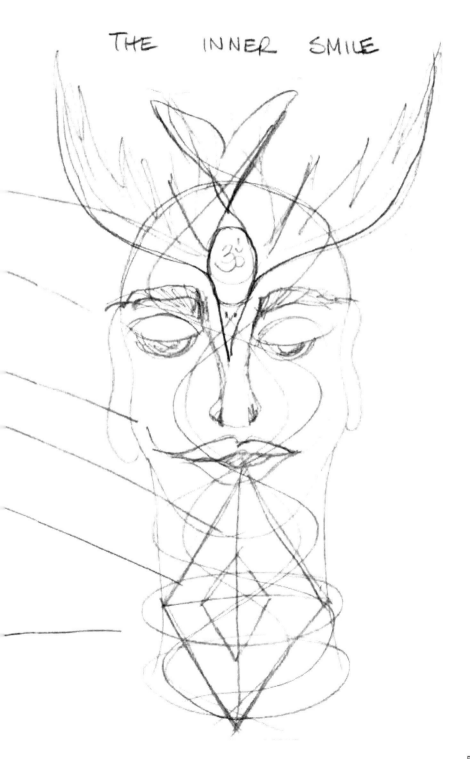

If the only words you ever say in prayer are "thank you," this is enough.

—Mother Teresa

Three Magic Wishes

In Yoga we say "be careful what you wish for
because you will get it."

I spent my teenage years pondering this,
for I knew intuitively,
my wishes would come true.

By age twenty, I had chosen
my three magic wishes.

In Greek we say "eeyia prota!"
Health first!

(1)
True Health
involves the whole
spiritual, psychological, emotional, and physical.

"Me eeyia olla yinoune."
With health, all is accomplished
and brings us Wealth.

(2)
True Wealth
begins with
profound
gratitude and appreciation
for the miraculous basics:
air, water, earth . . . sun, moon, stars,
and
awareness of it All.

And thus

(3)
True Happiness
arises
like the sun and moon
in a clear sky,
a light filled with love and joy
shared
with all of creation.

"Na eemaste panda agapimeni."
May we be always loved and loving.

What do you wish for?

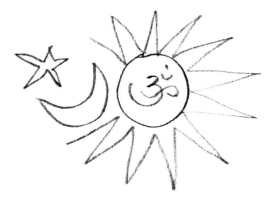

Simplicity of character
is the natural result
of profound thought.

—Chinese saying

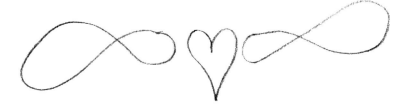

Love with all one's soul and
leave the rest to fate.

—Vladimir Nabokov

Letter to a Dying Friend

Spring 2003

Dearest Karen,

Please find enclosed a special candle of lavender for you
to light for your father. May your father's passing into the
Light be filled with Love and Peace.

A while ago, you asked me if I thought you would be
cured of cancer. I replied that yes, you have cancer, but that
I did not know what it meant to be cured. I have been
contemplating and reading since that conversation, and I
now have an answer:

To be cured is to be able to "heal that which remains
unloved and unloving."

Life is mysterious, and none of us knows when our time
comes to shed our physical bodies. Our physical body is a
burden, a beast of burden, and the best we can do is to
take care of our body and to love it like we do our beloved
pets. In the end, being allowed to shed our physical body
is a relief.

For me, spiritual practice has been the ongoing cultivation
of gratitude, compassion, understanding, and forgiveness—
both toward myself as well as all others. Practice has
helped me feel a Grace so profound that I can feel Infinite
Love in me, through me, and all around me. For me,
dying is being able to go back Home into the realm of
Infinite Love.

In the meantime, my human job as mother and daughter and sister and friend is the day-to-day practice of releasing the painful and confusing past in order to give and receive Love unconditionally.

Dearest Karen, our friendship is such a beautiful gift, truly a "feast for the heart." I feel our hearts are united in the journey of healing. Please allow the burning of this candle to also represent the letting go of the grief in our hearts that we may be free to Love in a big way.

I am so grateful the Universe has brought us each other.
You are so easy to love.
You are in my prayers and in my heart always.

Friends for Life and beyond.

With all my love,

angelA ♡

(Karen passed away shortly after,
just shy of her fiftieth birthday.)

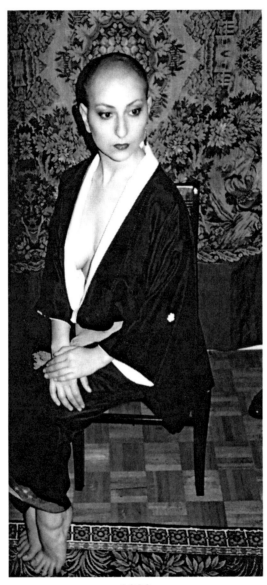

•1983•

Lead me from the unreal to the Real.
Lead me from darkness to Light.
Lead me from death to Immortality.

—Brihadaranyaka Upanishad

Epilogue

Yoga in the West has gone from being esoteric and on the
fringe to now being mainstream as a physical workout.

The physical practice of Yoga is merely
a means to the end.

In this book, we introduce the primary posture of *savasana*—
"corpse pose"—as the beginning point for inner work.

When the corpse comes back to life, it seeks freedom,
(in movement)
and there is a science for rising up
(into the sitting postures and into the standing postures).

I look forward to discussing and showing
the evolution of postures and inner work
in further works and mediums,
especially the visual.

Thank you for reading my book.

Please visit:
www.AlphaOmegaYoga.com
www.angelAKolias.com

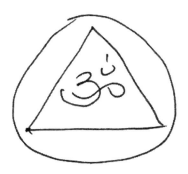

About the Author

Born May 15, 1960, in Calgary, Alberta, Canada, to
Greek immigrant parents, Greek was my first language.

Being baptized and raised in the Greek Orthodox Church was
a rich experience even though I was kicked out of Sunday
School as a precocious child of eight years old for
asking too many questions.

My spiritual search thus began by approaching
our various religious communities here
to talk to them and to read their literature.

By age twelve, I had settled in with the Jewish community,
studying weekly with the rabbi and taking Hebrew to
better understand the Scriptures. I also discovered
Kabbalah, but the rabbi told me I was considered too
young to study this with him.

At sixteen, my Jewish intellectual friends introduced me
to the concept of "voluntary simplicity"
and suggested I study Buddhism.
Thus began my shift into the Eastern philosophies.
At this time, I also became a top student in physics.
My love and study of physics is ongoing.

I began practicing Yoga at nineteen.

By twenty-one, I was enrolled in the University of Calgary
Religious Studies program, and my professors were
most supportive of my focus on Mysticism
as found throughout history in the various global
traditions, both Eastern and Western.

By age twenty-three, I was one of Alberta's first certified
yoga teachers with my own studio in Calgary called
Shiva Shakti.

On June 24, 1985, I gave birth to my daughter,
Sheika Luna Sol Chandra Mani Maria Ekaterina,
in my yoga studio without assistance.
I brought her out, a healthy eight-pound baby girl,
on my own while squatting
and then breast-fed her for almost three years.
She was truly a yoga baby.
Sheika Luna Sol is now married to a beautiful young man
and completing a teaching degree.

As an empty nester, I now have the time and space
for a new "baby." Thus, my first book—
which is written in "sutra" form and means "seeds"—
uses as few words as possible to give clues
to the Big Picture.

I hope you find my book interesting. I look forward to
sharing more in various mediums including the
audio and visual ones.

I wish you all lives filled with
love, light, health, beauty, and truth,
co-creating sacred space inside out:
heaven on earth.

Thank you.
angelA

AS ABOVE SO BELOW

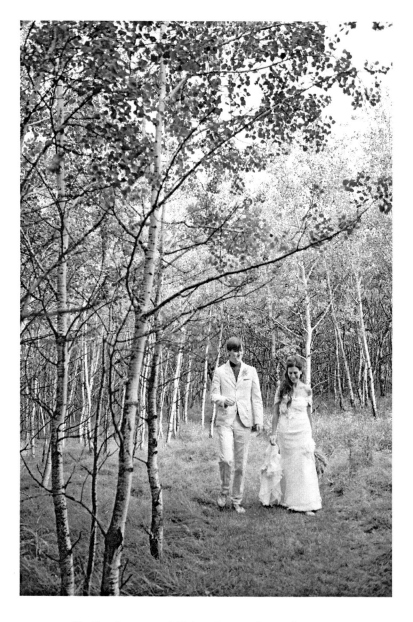

♥Sheika Luna and Kris - September 5th, 2010♥
photo: Dana Pugh

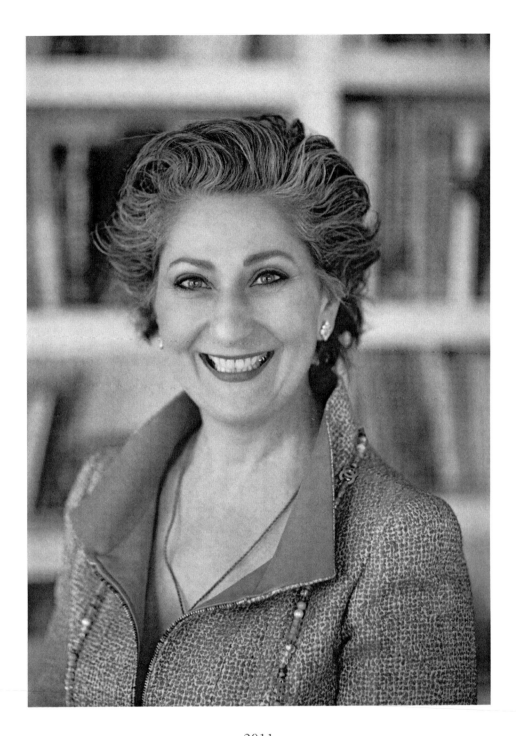

2011
photo: Gabe McClintock,   hair: Jerome

Afterword

Angela is available for speaking engagements
as well as for private consultations and sessions.

One of Angela's areas of focus is bringing practical mysticism
into the world of business where ethics and integrity are instrumental
in forming enhanced communities for living and working in.

Brought up in an entrepreneurial family
with real estate development on her father's side
and restaurants on her mother's side
economics truly began in the home.

Knowing how to run a house and family
with all the various responsibilities life requires
translates naturally to running businesses as well.

Angela is accomplished in the areas of
commercial multi-family real estate developments,
investments, finance and management.

In 2005 Angela married Kenneth Titcomb, a master chef.
Kenneth's two charming children, Christina, born 1984, and
Justin, born 1988, are now underwing and blooming beautifully.

Angela can be reached by email for further information:
angela@alphaomegayoga.com

References

I would like to share a short list of some of my favorites.

Campbell, Joseph with Bill Moyers. *The Power of Myth.* Betty Sue Flowers, ed. (Doubleday, New York, New York, 1988).

Crowley, Vivianne. *Thorson's Principles of Jungian Spirituality* (Thorson's, An Imprint of HarperCollins*Publishers*, Hammersmith, London, 1998).

Grey, Alex. *Sacred Mirrors: The Visionary Art of Alex Grey* (Inner Traditions International, Rochester, Vermont, 1990).

Hay, Louise L. *Heal Your Body: The Mental Causes for Physical Illness and the Metaphysical Way to Overcome Them* (Hay House, Inc., United States, 1988).

Iyengar, B.K.S., *Light on Life: The Yoga Journey to Wholeness, Inner Peace, and Ultimate Freedom* (Raincoast Books, Vancouver, Canada, 2005).

Iyengar, Geeta S. *Yoga: A Gem for Women* (Allied Publishers Private Limited, New Delhi, 1987)

Jung, C.G., *The Collected Works, Volume 14: Mysterium Coniunctionis; An Inquiry into the Seperation and Synthesis of Psychic Opposites in Alchemy.* Trans. R. F. C Hull. (Bollingen Series XX, Princeton University Press, Princeton, N.J., 1989).

Kingsley, Peter. *Ancient Philosophy, Mystery, and Magic: Empedocles and Pythagorean Tradition* (Clarendon Press, Oxford University Press Inc., New York, 1995).

Kingsley, Peter. *Reality* (The Golden Sufi Center, Point Reyes, California, 2010).

Regardie, Isreal. *The Art of True Healing* (Helios Book Service (Publications) Ltd., Cheltenham, Glos., 1966).

Kingston, Karen. *Clear Your Clutter with Feng Shui* (Broadway Books, New York, 1999).

Mitchell, Stephen. *Tao Te Ching: A New English Version* (HarperPerennial ModemClassics, New York, 2006).

Radha, Swami Sivananda. *The Yoga of Healing* (Timeless Books, B.C., Canada and Spokane, Washington, 2007).

Radha, Swami Sivananda. *The Divine Light Invocation: A Healing Meditation* (Timeless Books, B.C., Canada and Spokane, Washington, 2001).

Sternberg, Esther M., M.D., *Healing Spaces: The Science of Place and Well-Being* (The Belknap Press of Harvard University Press, Cambridge, Massachusetts, 2010).

Suzuki, Shunryu. *Zen Mind, Beginner's Mind.* Trudy Dixon, ed. (John Weatherhill, Inc., New York, N.Y., 1977).

Tolle, Eckhart. *A New Earth: Awakening to Your Life's Purpose* (Penguin Group, USA, 2005).

Watts, Alan W. *Nature, Man and Woman* (Vintage Books, A Division of Random House, Inc., New York, 1991).

Watts, Alan W. *The Philosophies of Asia: the Edited Transcripts* (Charles. E. Tuttle Company, Inc. of Rutland, Vermont, 1995).

Wells, HG. *The Outline of History* (Doubleday & Company, Inc., Garden City, New York, 1971).

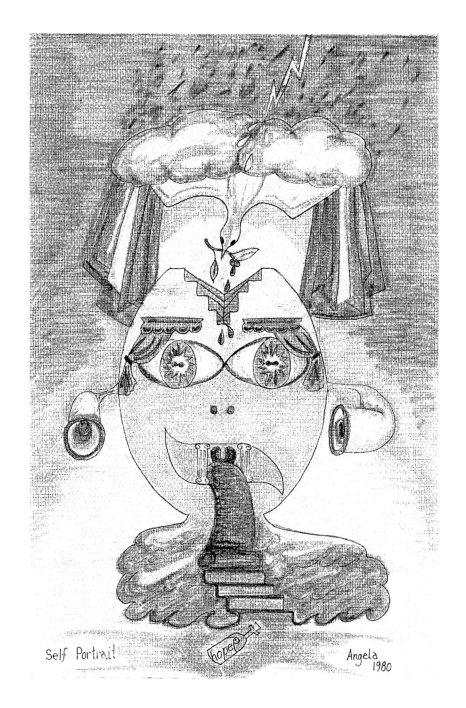

OPEN MIND
Self Portrait at age 19

Notes

Notes

CPSIA information can be obtained at www.ICGtesting.com
Printed in the USA
LVOW041517140512

281675LV00004B/129/P

9 781462 856305